At Peace With Food

Leeann Simons, MS, RD, LDN
Nutritionist

ISBN: 1-4392-2372-6
ISBN-13: 9781439223727

Visit www.booksurge.com to order additional copies.

TABLE OF CONTENTS

Dedication· ii

Introduction · 1

Chapter 1: Why Me?· · · · · · · · · · · · · · · · · · 5

Chapter 2: Why Don't Diets Work?· · · · · · · · · · · · · ·11

Chapter 3: Diet Contradictions and Consequences · · · · · ·19

Chapter 4: The Metabolic March Backwards · · · · · · · · ·31

Chapter 5: Fear of Food Freedom · · · · · · · · · · · · ·41

Chapter 6: The Food Court of Law· · · · · · · · · · · · · 49

Chapter 7: Three Rules of Thumb · · · · · · · · · · · · · ·57

Chapter 8: About Weight Control · · · · · · · · · · · · · 65

Chapter 9: Learning to Be a Healthy Eater · · · · · · · · · · 77

The End, and a New Beginning: Making the Relationship
Work · 85

Dedication

To my dad: it ain't radio, but it will have to do

To Jan: OK lady, it's your turn

To Daryl: thank you, for everything

NOTE: Information in this book should NEVER replace any medical advice you have received from your primary care doctor or other medical professionals

Introduction

☒ **What diet is going to work for me?**

☒ **Which is the best diet?**

☒ **Why isn't my diet working?**

☒ **How come I can be successful at my job but I can't be successful losing weight?**

☒ **What's wrong with me?**

These are only some of the questions I've heard throughout my years as a registered dietitian. They are all good questions, with no one answer. Truthfully? I don't have a single answer to these questions, and that is why I started on this journey to figure out how to help people lose weight—without dieting.

Have you asked yourself any of these questions? The last one is the most important, you know. You should always get a physical to rule out medical causes, but in most cases there is nothing physically wrong. There *is*, however, something wrong with dieting.

By the time you're finished reading this, I hope you'll be able to glimpse what your life could be like if you stopped dieting and started losing weight. My hope is that you will be able to allow yourself the freedom to get rid of the burden of diets and learn how to become *At Peace with Food*.

Are You Ready?

Now you must ask yourself: Are you ready to give up dieting forever? Are you ready to learn to accept your body, whatever shape you may currently be in? Can you learn to have a normal relationship with food?

Please understand that being *At Peace with Food* is not going to work for everyone—but not just for medical reasons. You have to be willing to take the risk of overeating and learning to listen to your body. In many cases, it is learning to listen for the first time in many, many years, because you have been programmed to eat for a variety of reasons, the least of which is time of day and "cleaning your plate." Not everyone is ready to pay attention to him- or herself in such a personal way. Most of us are quite comfortable with structure: it's what we have grown up with, and it's what we know. Giving up the known for the unknown is scary.

So you must really want to give up dieting forever. You must be willing to take that risk. It's not just for a day. It's not just for a week. It's forever. And from personal experience, let me just say that if this works for you, you may find it to be one of the most freeing, liberating experiences you've ever had.

Are you ready? Come on—you know you are!

Chapter 1: Why Me?

What qualifies me to write about this topic? Let me tell you a bit about myself. My name is Leeann Simons, and I have been a registered dietitian for over twenty-five years. This means that I have worked with hundreds of clients in various settings, including hospitals, doctor's offices, sports facilities, and privately (sometimes even meeting at a coffee shop). It's always satisfying to be able to help people with their nutrition issues, ranging from high cholesterol to diabetes to most often (and many times related to the previous conditions) weight. But diet and nutrition can also be very frustrating, as I am sure you know.

I certainly know, because in addition to being a registered dietitian, I also used to be about twenty-five pounds overweight. I'll tell you more about that later, but for now let me just say that it wasn't until I stopped dieting that I finally started losing weight—and keeping it off.

In addition to working with individuals, I also teach a science of nutrition class at a business school. Perhaps surprisingly, my class is one of the most popular electives. I spend a lot of time teaching my students to be good consumers, read labels, and make choices regarding nutrition. The most fun for me, though, are the questions they ask. And wouldn't you know that one of the most popular questions is "what is the best diet?"

I used to answer this question by saying very firmly, "Diets don't work. Forget them, period." But over time I have come to realize that I lose people's attention pretty quickly when I say that. Now I tell folks, "All diets work—while you're on them. The proof is in the maintenance."

What Makes Me Think I'm the Expert?

"Leeann," you may be asking me, "what makes you so qualified to tell *me* how to lose weight? You're a registered dietitian, so you know about diets, but what do you really know about *me*?"

This is a wonderful question, and one I love to answer. It's simple: I've been there. No, I've never been obese, so I don't know if this type of lifestyle change works for people in that situation. I do believe, however, that since diets don't work, the non-dieting approach to weight loss is where we must focus. Certainly, if you have a particular health condition (such as diabetes or kidney disease), you need to be more focused about what you eat, and you definitely want a closer relationship with a dietitian to meet your nutrition needs, so this may not be the best option for you.

But for everyone who wants to lose those twenty-five or thirty pounds, *I have been there*. About twenty-five years ago, I used to weigh twenty-five or thirty pounds (depending on the day and time of the month, of course) more than I do now.

I always thought of myself as overweight. When I was a teenager, hot pants were the style. I may have looked good in hot pants for one afternoon, but I'm just not genetically predisposed to have thin thighs. And when the media tells you what's in style, if you don't look good in it, it's not the style; it's you. Looking at pictures of myself from my high school days, I see that I was not overweight. I was fine. But I never really had any reinforcement to make me feel that way.

Then I went to college and gained the freshmen ten. I remember going to the dining halls and getting huge salads with this marvelous cottage cheese dressing. I remember thinking, *This must be good for me because it's cottage cheese*, so I loaded it onto the salad. I never knew the dressing was also loaded with mayonnaise.

My first summer after college I was an assistant baker at a camp, and I put on another ten or fifteen pounds. When you're making fifty loaves of bread three times a day, half a loaf right out of the oven, dripping with butter, will never be missed by anyone—certainly my body (especially my waist and thighs) didn't miss out on it, or the extra weight that I kept on for several more years.

So I began to diet. My "diet history" includes the Scarsdale Diet (anyone remember that?), the Atkins Diet, Weight Watchers, starch blockers (the little pills that were supposed to allow you to eat as much bread, cereal, and pasta as you wanted and never gain weight)—you name it, pretty much whatever was out there, I tried.

I remember buying a book describing how fasting would rid my body of toxins crawling under my skin as a result of my horrendous food choices. Think about that for a minute! How do you feel when you are told your body is a chemical waste dump? First of all, it's not true; and secondly, it is never a good thing to think of your body as terminally poisonous! How can you get out of bed in the morning with such a sentence over your head?

However, I thought this was what I needed to do, because I *did* believe what the book said. And, of course, I never made it past the first twelve hours of fasting.

What about those money back guarantees? I was too embarrassed to let anyone know I'd failed. I remember those weekly Weight Watchers meetings, one of the many times I joined. Let me

Preface by saying to those of you to whom this program has worked—that's great. It is one of the more "fair and balanced" programs out there for people who like them. For me, though, it was a dismal failure. I would fast the day of the meeting (which was always at night), weigh in, and then go out and eat, figuring I had a whole other week to lose weight.

So I have been there.

What finally worked for me was giving up dieting. I just stopped. I remember walking with a friend around what used to be the golf course at Penn State, where I was attending graduate school for nutrition science. We were talking about what it could be like if we could eat whatever we wanted, whenever we wanted. We discussed what the impact could be not only on our bodies but more importantly on our minds, emotions, and sense of self.

We'd been reading a wonderful book by Susan Orbach called *Fat Is a Feminist Issue II* . This book described a world where women ate whatever they wanted, whenever they wanted. It discussed what happened to people when they allowed themselves to enjoy food and let go of all the rules about "healthy eating." Yes, these women gained weight; but then, as food lost its power, they stopped eating all the time and began *losing* weight.

Yes, you might go kind of crazy at first, of course. But over time what happens is that food loses its power to make or break your self-image. If you can eat those cookies whenever you want, suddenly you don't feel the need to eat as many, or as often. The first few times you may eat the whole box and get sick. But over time you learn to listen to your hunger. You may only be hungry for two cookies, and you learn how to be satisfied.

When I began to think about trying this, believe me, it was quite scary. It sounded so new, so different, and so wonderful—but I was afraid. What if I couldn't stop myself from eating? What if I "gave myself permission" all the time, and I just kept putting on more and more weight? It was, truly, a risk.

But it was also one of the most liberating experiences of my life. And it worked. I have kept that weight off, plus or minus a pound or two, for over twenty-five years.

Now I ask your permission to take the opportunity to help those of you who may have experiences similar to mine learn to do this for yourselves. It's a risky proposition to give up all that fear, power, and emotion associated with food. But let me work with you, and together we can work on giving up the dieting mentality, learning how to enjoy eating again, and becoming *At Peace with Food*.

Chapter 2: Why Don't Diets Work?

Regardless of what diet you choose, whether it's nutritionally balanced (such as Weight Watchers and parts of the South Beach Diet) or just off the wall (the Cabbage Soup Diet, the Vinegar and Honey Cleanse), they *all* work—while you are on them. You are highly motivated, excited about new changes you see in your future, and you have very high expectations of what's going to happen with your new body.

Yet, eventually, whether it's two hours, a day, a month, or six months, you go off the diet. And then? The weight returns, often bringing company in the form of additional pounds, resulting in a higher weight than you had at the beginning of your diet.

Think of the behaviors that lead you to overeating. Do you eat when you're under stress? Studying for an exam? When you are sad? Angry? When you go on a diet, what you are doing is giving up control of your eating behaviors to someone (or something) else. This means you're not responsible for your food choices. Taking away that responsibility makes life a lot easier for many people, especially those trying to lose weight. If you're not responsible for your food choices and something goes wrong, it's not your fault, right? Wrong.

The thing is, I'm not talking about responsibility for paying the bills, picking up the laundry, or walking the dog. I'm talking about the responsibility for eating foods that affect your weight and, more importantly, your health (both mental and physical).

So, you go on this diet, follow this plan, all the while not addressing the underlying behaviors that lead to your overeating. Let's say the diet goes very well and you lose twenty or thirty pounds. Once you reach your goal (and that's assuming you didn't get frustrated and quit dieting after three hours), then what? What happens when you find yourself in a stressful situation? Your boss gives you a task you find too difficult, you flunk an exam, your spouse looks at you the wrong way. If you haven't figured out how to deal with the underlying causes of your food issues, when you find yourself back in one of those situations, you will find yourself going back to your old behavior—eating.

Not figuring out what caused you to overeat to begin with, and not changing that behavior, is one of the most important reasons why diets don't work.

Another reason is that we tend to set unrealistic goals. We raise our expectations for how life will be once the weight is gone—expectations that often are impossible to meet. For example, *I am going to lose twenty pounds by the end of the month, get into a size three dress* (is there such a thing as size three?)*, and find myself a wonderful job and a new boyfriend.*

How do those goals sound? Not just one, but *three* goals! And we haven't even mentioned world peace and feeding the hungry.

Let's look at a fitness analogy. If you never jogged, would you start out running twenty miles the day you bought your new, expensive sneakers? I surely hope not. You might never be able to move your legs again! Hopefully, you would find out how to start a realistic plan to break in those sneakers (and not your feet). You would start slowly, perhaps alternating between walking for a minute and jogging for half a minute, and over time build up to eventually meet your long-term goal, whatever it might be.

The same is true for weight control. We tend to set the rung too high and it becomes impossible to reach. If you think you can lose twenty pounds in a month, and you're five days into your diet and have only lost two pounds—well, you'll never reach your goal, so why continue dieting? Why bother trying? You'll never make it, and sadly, you'll wind up thinking about food and failure all the time.

Why Am I So Bad When I'm Trying to Be So Good?

It was Erma Bombeck who first used the phrase "guilt is the gift that keeps on giving." I'm not sure she realized that it applied not just to behaviors surrounding caring and giving but also to eating. I happen to think this is particularly appropriate for folks trying to lose weight. If you think about what happens when you think you've been "bad" (and I'll get to that in a minute), you feel guilty. And this guilt? It's like the never ending math equation—it just keeps multiplying and multiplying. You feel like you've failed, so what happens to your motivation to change your behavior? It disappears. You ask yourself, *Why should I change if I'm only going to fail?* And then what happens? You feel the need to punish yourself. And how do you do that? By continuing to eat.

That's why this "bad" label drives me crazy. Every time people tell me, "I was bad," in reference to their diets, I want to shoot them just to show them what "bad" really is. It's ridiculous! I meet people all the time—wonderful, successful people who like their jobs, their families, just about everything about their lives except their diets. And because of this, they consider themselves to be failures. They've been able to meet so many goals, at work, at home, in sports. But they would give up all their successes if they could only attain this one goal: to lose weight.

Let me tell you a story about one of these people I saw as a client. She came into my office looking at the floor, as if she were ashamed. We exchanged our hellos, and I asked how she was doing. Slowly she looked up at me and said, "I was bad."

I heard myself ask, "Did you rob a bank?" She shook her head negatively. "Did you shoot someone?" Again, no. So I asked her what possibly could have happened to make her so sad, and she said, "I ate three pieces of birthday cake at my daughter's party."

Why is it that people place judgments on their eating behaviors? People are "good" or "bad" based on what they've eaten? That sounds crazy, doesn't it? Don't you think people are good or bad based on, well, whether they've robbed a bank? Hit their child? Voted for the other candidate, at least!

Stop feeling bad and guilty about food! Instead, take a moment and try the following:

Imagine what it feels like to *not* feel guilty after eating dessert. You just ate a lovely chocolate torte for the sheer pleasure of eating. You allowed yourself to enjoy the smell, the taste, and the texture of this delectable item. Without the guilt, how do you feel?

You feel great! Without the guilt you have no reason to "punish" yourself and you can move forward with your life because without the guilt you can be *At Peace with Food.*

So please, stop placing judgment on what you eat or don't eat. Save the "bad" label for when you shoot someone.

Don't *Should* On Yourself

Many years ago, I was sitting with my good friend Jan, discussing strategies for working with clients to help them meet their weight and exercise goals. She had discovered that one of the major stumbling blocks preventing success was her clients' overwhelming sense of guilt. It wasn't that they were unable to follow a specific plan for eating, or that they didn't like exercise. Those things were sometimes part of it, but the main factor was that as a result of not being able to meet their goals they felt they had failed because they didn't do what they "should" be doing.

Because her clients were constantly telling her, "I should eat better, I should exercise more, I should not have had those cookies, I am a bad person," she came up with this wonderful phrase: Don't *should* on yourself. Isn't that a wonderful piece of advice? Of course, you must watch how you say it (try repeating it three times fast and you'll see what I mean); yet when stated slowly and clearly, it does cover a lot of ground.

Think about it for a moment. What do you experience when you think you haven't done the things you *should* have done? How do you feel when you didn't meet your exercise goal for the week? When you didn't lose all the weight you thought you should? Probably not good. Why do you think this is true? Usually it's because you've set yourself one of those unrealistic goals (run five miles every day and never eat chocolate again) that are impossible to meet. And when you are unable to meet your goal, you feel terrible.

For some reason, while we often say, "patience is a virtue," we are unable to apply it to very personal situations, such as improving our health by losing weight and beginning to exercise. We set amazingly unrealistic goals (lose twenty-five pounds, run the marathon) and expect to be able to accomplish these goals yesterday. We set impossibly high expectations for ourselves. Then, when we realize we cannot possibly live up to these expectations, we conclude we have failed, never having seen that failure was the only outcome we could have expected.

When you are *At Peace with Food*, and at peace with yourself, you find that the decisions you make about your health are more realistic. You learn to move more slowly, realizing that you are not in a race to become healthy. Rather, you're developing a new relationship with yourself, and new relationships, if they are to be good ones, take time. You learn to set realistic goals, starting off slowly and building up.

You learn how to change behaviors because you realize you want to, not because you *should*.

Chapter 3: Diet Contradictions and Consequences

Too Many Diets, Too Many Calories

What, you may ask, is a diet contradiction? Think about the last time you went to the supermarket. Can you count on one hand the number of diet foods available (fat free, carbohydrate free, low calorie—you get the idea)? Two hands? Twelve? We have more and more sugar free products, more and more diet books—and what's the result? An obesity epidemic.

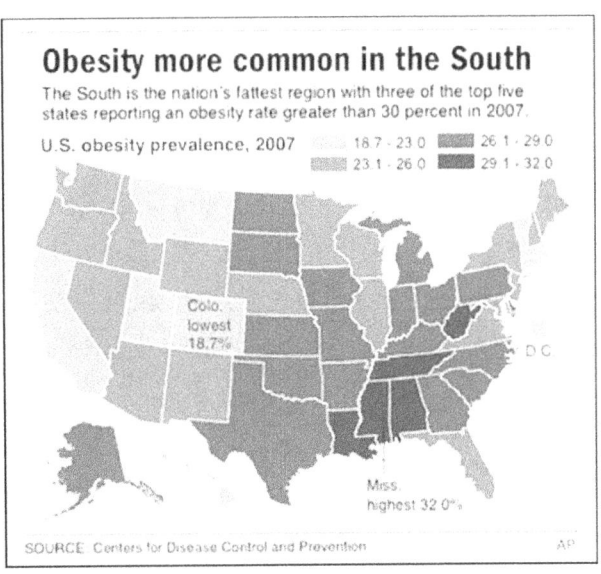

Obesity more common in the South

The South is the nation's fattest region with three of the top five states reporting an obesity rate greater than 30 percent in 2007.

U.S. obesity prevalence, 2007
- 18.7 - 23.0
- 23.1 - 26.0
- 26.1 - 29.0
- 29.1 - 32.0

Colo. lowest 18.7%

D.C.

Miss. highest 32.0%

SOURCE: Centers for Disease Control and Prevention   AP

This "map," in the July 18, 2008, *Washington Post*, shows the contradiction. While the article discusses how the South has the highest level of obesity, it also reminds us that despite all the efforts being made to encourage us to lose weight, the number of adults in the United States who are obese has increased between 2005 and 2007.

How is this possible? The article does discuss how poverty forces people to make poor choices: fast food is cheaper and comes in supersizes. Economics does indeed play a role for many people when it comes to food selection. But what about people for whom money is not a consideration?

With all these extra diet products on the shelves, you'd think we'd be thinner and healthier, not needing to concern ourselves with disease. Instead, we're finding an increase in what are called "obesity related diseases." One such disease is Type 2 diabetes. (This is the diabetes associated with extra weight and obesity, not the type related to the pancreas' inability to produce insulin, the hormone necessary to absorb sugar.) We also find an increase in high blood pressure, or hypertension, and an increase in heart disease. What's most disturbing is that these conditions are being found in younger and younger individuals. Prescriptions for medications to treat these diseases in adults are now being written for children, and we have no idea what the long-term implications will be. But health care providers are concerned with what they are seeing *now*, concerned that they cannot wait for the research.

In addition to obesity related diseases, we see, quite paradoxically, an increase in eating disorders. It is the obsession with food that leads not only to eating disorders (like anorexia and bulimia) but also to **disordered eating**—an inability to have a healthy relationship with our diets and our bodies.

Most of us know what an **eating disorder** is: eating disorders have a medical diagnosis based on a specific set of criteria (e.g. bulimia involves recurrent episodes of binge eating followed by compensatory behaviors, such as vomiting and abuse of laxatives and/or enemas, with the thought of preventing weight gain).

Disordered eating, on the other hand, includes a wide range of behaviors from dieting, binging, and purging to fasting to chewing and spitting. These behaviors can be part of an eating disorder, but by themselves are not diagnostic of one.

We all may periodically display some disordered behaviors, but it is their repeated occurrence under certain circumstances that may ultimately result in the out-of-control symptoms of an eating disorder.

As a registered dietitian, I feel that my profession has inadvertently contributed to the development of these conditions. One of the dietitian's jobs has been to tell people how to eat. We give people menus, figure out calorie requirements, and then follow up with our clients, congratulating them when they meet their goals and sharing disappointment when goals aren't met.

There is no cure for eating disorders, no one treatment that works for every person (that "one size fits all" mentality). Each person comes to this diagnosis with her (or, increasingly, his) own history, and treatment must be developed accordingly. A colleague of mine, Trisha Gura, has written a wonderful book, *Lying in Weight*, that has helped her deal with her own situation as an adult who suffered with anorexia. She looks at eating disorders as a chronic illness, one that may go into remission for long periods of time but that under stressful circumstances may reappear.

Another author, Kim Chernin, wrote of her experiences with her eating disorder and recovery in *The Obsession-Reflections on the Tyranny of Slenderness*. She writes of her awakening to what was causing her episodes of binging and what she discovered as she was began to resume control over her behaviors:

"For many weeks after that time I found that whenever I was in conflict about food what I needed was permission to eat. If I was in fact able to let myself eat for pleasure, the terrible conflict abated and with it the sense of an insatiable hunger. Frequently, as I observed this conflict over food, I noticed that the permission to eat was closely linked to a delight in life, a sense of joy and abundance, an awareness of some unexpected meaning or beauty. And, frequently, too, there were memories of childhood. Occasionally, walking down the street with a salted pretzel from the street stand at the edge of the college campus, I would feel that I had little legs and hands, that I was walking in the Bronx with my mother, tasting everything for the first time. In this state of delight, it never took a great deal of food to satisfy my hunger. However plain or simple it was, to me it seemed exactly the pleasure and satisfaction I had been looking for. The moral to draw from this seemed clear. There was a state of mind and being in which food became a simple uncomplicated sensual pleasure. But if I

> were lacking this state, if I simply could not give myself permission to eat, food would not satisfy me, no matter how excellent it was, or how much of it I consumed in compulsive rebellion again my own prohibition."

This "giving of permission" sounds an awful lot like becoming *At Peace with Food*, doesn't it?

And so, as I said earlier, we have this paradox: increasing incidence of anorexia and bulimia paralleling an obesity epidemic.

What's wrong with this picture? Not only are we being bombarded with diet products while finding ourselves getting fatter, but we are also being given next to impossible guidelines (orders?) for exercise. It seems different every week: an hour a day, thirty minutes three times a week—what next? You feel like you have to exercise, exercise, exercise. Then you have to reduce, reduce, reduce your intake of the foods you like, reducing the pleasures you have with eating.

While all this is happening, what's increasing may not only be your weight but also your self-loathing. While you're trying to achieve some "ideal" weight goal, your only success appears to be in not liking yourself. We're being given unrealistic orders and setting unrealistic expectations for ourselves, and then we're surprised when these goals cannot be met.

I hope my profession is changing. I know that the people I work with have. We no longer feel the need to tell people what to do (unless there is a specific medical condition requiring specific guidelines, as in kidney or liver disease). We now try to find out exactly what the person wants to do, meet them at the point, and work with them to set realistic goals.

Later in this book I will give you a "prescription" for starting an activity program, with small attainable goals, so don't fret—help is here.

The Last Supper

Let's look at a few of the things you may be giving up while learning to become *At Peace with Food*. And, as always, let me start by sharing a personal story with you.

This experience occurred only a few years ago, long after I'd given up dieting. The Atkins Diet—you know, the low carbohydrate diet—was suddenly back in the press, *big time*. It was in all the papers and all the movie stars were doing it after they had gained weight for this movie or that film, so everyone was jumping back on the bandwagon (for a diet that's been around over thirty years.)

First, I'd like to say that one of the positive results of the reemergence of this diet is that it is now being studied in a scientific manner, like many other diets. The results of the studies are surprising: Atkins eating doesn't increase heart disease or blood cholesterol, as originally thought. Of course, the plan now recommends more plant-based proteins, instead of bacon and sausage, but the results are still surprising.

However, it is still a diet. And further results of these studies continue to show that most of the weight that is lost occurs in the first six months, and most may be gained back after two years.

So we see proof of the first consequence of dieting—the weight returns.

Based on the renewed popularity of the Atkins diet, I decided to go on this diet for two weeks. I would keep scrupulous records, watch my weight carefully (obsessively, it turned out, albeit for a short time), give up all carbohydrates, and in addition to the food records, record how I felt in a mood journal. And then I would write an article for the *American Journal of Clinical Nutrition*, the professional journal for dietitians. Think of it—a "real" dietitian, dieting and reporting the results. I thought it would be quite an exciting thing to do.

Then I realized I would have to give up cappuccino, because it contains the dietary carbohydrate lactose. That made me second-guess whether or not this was such a good idea, but my husband said to me, "Look, you're only talking two weeks. Don't make such a big deal." He might not have understood my love of cappuccino, but, I realized, this *was* research. People had given up much more for research. So I decided to go ahead with it for the greater good.

Guess what happened next? I bet you know. I went into "pre-diet" mode, which I hadn't done for years. I became obsessed with food. I went out and ate all kinds of things I knew I wasn't going to be able to eat for the next two weeks (and only two weeks!). It had been years since I'd gone into this "Last Supper" mode. Somewhere, in my subconscious, however, I knew I wasn't going to be able to eat certain foods, so I knew I had to have them—and I had to have them *now*.

Then I bought all types of high protein, high fat foods for the diet. Let me tell you, it wasn't easy. Growing up in a kosher home and then becoming a dietitian makes it difficult to buy bacon and sausage. But I bought lots of eggs, cheese, and herring in cream sauce. I also bought the "keto" sticks, which you put in your urine to see if you are in ketosis (a metabolic state that happens when your body has no carbohydrate stores and begins burning fat). And I began the Atkins diet.

Two days, folks, I lasted two days. I hated obsessing about what I was going to eat, I didn't feel well, and *I didn't lose weight!* Now, *that* bothered me. From everything I'd read, everyone I'd spoken to, I should have been losing weight immediately. (See? I, too, was buying into the hype about quick weight loss!) I wasn't being at all realistic, considering my overeating the day before the diet began, but I wanted to believe—me, the registered dietitian with the knowledge why and how these things don't work.

When I reflect back on the experience, I realize that it didn't matter how much knowledge I had. I was back in Diet World, and all I could think about was losing weight.

Since I know myself, I realized that staying on this diet was not going to work, so I went off it. I didn't get to write that article for the nutrition journal. But I did get further confirmation that dieting doesn't work for me, and it doesn't work for a lot of other people, either.

Now, let's talk about you. How do you feel before you start dieting? Think about it for a few minutes—better yet, write it down. You need to think about how you feel when you know you're going to start depriving your body of foods you like. After all, for most of us, diet means deprivation, right? It's not exactly a gift you give yourself when you decide to go on a diet, is it?

Do you go into "Last Supper" mode? Many times this is referred to as the "Sunday Night Supper" because the most popular days for starting the new diet are, you guessed it, Mondays.

Understand that when you go on a diet, you will eventually go off the diet. I'm not sure this is what diet authors had in mind when they designed their diets, but we have learned that when folks go "on" a diet, the unfortunate but logical conclusion is that they eventually go "off" it. That's why nowadays you may hear advertisements for "lifestyle changes." Even diet promoters know that diets don't work. They are simply repackaged as these "lifestyle changes." As I said earlier, unless you change those *behaviors* that lead you to overeat to begin with, when you go off your diet, you will be back at the beginning—or worse.

Try to figure out what is making you want to eat. Think about what is leading you to these eating behaviors. Anger? Fear? Sadness? You must learn to reject that diet mentality! When you forget about dieting, you can start concentrating on the things that are really "eating" you and causing you to turn towards the chips and chocolate. *This* is the point where you need to start making changes.

Chapter 4: The Metabolic March Backwards

Have you heard of the "yo-yo" syndrome? This is what happens when you go on and off diets and your weight cycles down and up, and down…and up. The reality is that when you lose weight too quickly (which often happens with fad diets—you know, the ones that sound too good to be true, and usually are), some of that weight loss is indeed fat, which is good. But a lot of it is water and some of it is muscle tissue. So you do lose *weight*, but you aren't losing only *fat*. What happens when you ditch the diet and start eating again is that the weight comes back, but this time mostly as fat. So you not only wind up gaining more weight than you lost, you gain more fat. This changes what is called your *body composition* (the percent of body fat tissue as compared to muscle tissue). And this increase in body fat changes your metabolism for the worse.

Metabolism refers to the rate at which your body burns calories. People who have a higher percentage of muscle mass tend to have an easier time losing weight, and keeping it off, because muscle is what we call a more "metabolically active" tissue. It takes more calories to maintain muscle. Fat, however, tends to be kind of lazy. It doesn't take a lot of calories to keep it on, and once it's there it likes to stay put.

So, when your weight goes up and down, up and down, especially when you are losing some of that "metabolically active" muscle tissue, your body composition changes to not only result in more fat but less muscle, making your metabolism slow down. When your metabolism is slow, it becomes more difficult to lose weight.

It's not fair, but it's what happens.

Our bodies are uniquely designed to try, at all costs, to survive. During times of famine, the folks with the most fat are able to survive the longest off those fat stores. Fortunately, for most of us, famine is not something we are likely to experience in our lifetime. Unfortunately, many of us have bodies that would survive for a long time in that famine.

When you are depriving your body of the calories it needs by severely restricting your intake, your system doesn't know whether you are in Boston or Biafra, whether this fast is voluntary or involuntary. It doesn't know when the next meal is coming, or if it's ever going to get there. Therefore, it's going to conserve every single calorie it gets. The idea is survival—to provide your brain and central nervous system with whatever nutrients they need in order to keep you alive.

How does the body perform this magical feat of survival? By slowing down the rate at which it burns calories. In other words, by reducing your metabolic rate. Burning calories at a much slower rate allows your brain and central nervous system to keep functioning.

You don't have to be on a seriously restrictive diet for your metabolism to move into this mode, either. There's another common eating behavior that triggers this slowdown—skipping meals. We've all done it. We eat a lot at night and aren't hungry when we wake up. (Hmm, sounds like a Last Supper behavior). So we skip breakfast, thinking it will help us burn those extra calories we ate last night.

Think again.

When you skip a meal, you not only affect your metabolism, you unconsciously set yourself up to overeat later. Let's face it, six to eight hours is a long time to go without eating (even longer if it's breakfast you skipped). What happens is that by the time you "allow" yourself to eat, you're subconsciously thinking, *I didn't eat lunch, so I saved all sorts of calories and I can eat more for dinner*. Instead of having a four-ounce steak with a potato and salad, you order the twelve-ounce steak, mashed potatoes with butter, and a salad with creamy dressing. Why not? You haven't eaten all day, right?

Wrong. If you were consuming the amount of calories your body needed for weight loss, over time your body would lose that weight. But because you have gotten into the habit of skipping meals, when you finally eat you are consuming more calories than if you had eaten regularly throughout the day.

Now that I've (hopefully) chastised you into never skipping meals again, I want you to think about the cost of calorie restriction. No, I don't mean financially, and not even physically this time. I mean emotionally. What does dieting do to you emotionally?

First of all, you become obsessed with dieting. You become obsessed with getting that weight off, and you lose sight of what normal eating behaviors are. You no longer enjoy your relationship with food (if you ever had one), and this is bad.

Listen: life is short, and food should be just a *part* of what you think about. It's time to develop a new relationship with food. Instead of being marked by frustration and disappointment, by fear and competition between you and what you eat, food needs to take its place as one of the many activities in your life, along with family, friends, working, and being active. And, like these other activities, it should be pleasurable.

Another emotional "side-effect" of a diet prescription is increased self-doubt. Too many times my clients have told me they no longer think they can make healthy choices for themselves. Not only do they doubt their ability to make healthy decisions, they no longer trust themselves. Dieting causes them to feel like they've lost the ability to make correct choices for a healthy body—choices that *do* include "forbidden foods." Think about it: when you stop dieting, no food is forbidden!

The Biology of Human Starvation

Let me tell you about a landmark study by Dr. Ancel Keyes, published in 1950 in the book *The Biology of Human Starvation*. It became famous because it provided the military with information on what occurred to refugees and POWs in Europe during World War II. Its results still resonate today because of the eerie comparisons seen between the starving men in 1944 and what happens with people who decide to voluntarily starve themselves to lose weight for personal reasons.

In 1944, thirty-six healthy male subjects volunteered to participate in an experiment designed to copy the starvation conditions of war-torn Europe as World War II was coming to an end. These men were conscientious objectors, who felt that while they would not fight in the war they could contribute to the war effort by helping to learn what was happening to the millions of people suffering from starvation in Europe.

The results became known as the Minnesota Starvation Experiment, the Minnesota Semi-Starvation Experiment, and the Starvation Study. This grueling research was designed to help researchers gain an understanding of the biological and psychological effects of semi-starvation and the problems of re-feeding the surviving civilians as well as returning prisoners of war. While the results of the study were not published in time to help with World War II survivors, they give us interesting insight into what happens to the body under starvation conditions.

Dr. Keyes and his colleagues interviewed many young men for their physical as well as psychological stamina. They then chose thirty-six who were healthy physically and mentally. For the first three months they collected baseline data; the men were fed diets similar to what they would eat under normal, healthy circumstances, around 3500 calories a day. The next six months were referred to as the "semi-starvation" portion of the study. This consisted of about 1500-1800 calories a day, with foods similar to what refugees and POWs might have received in Europe (mostly carbohydrates—potatoes, bread, turnips). The subjects were also expected to perform daily assigned tasks, as well as walk around twenty miles per week (as a POW might be forced to do). During this time, most of the volunteers lost up to 25 percent of their weight.

The final three months were the re-feeding portion of the study, also known as nutritional rehabilitation. Their diets were not restricted, but what they ate was carefully recorded (along with their behaviors).

What happened to these men was astounding. Along with losing up to 25 percent of their body weight, the psychological, emotional, and physical changes found during and after the study are strikingly similar to those we see in today's chronic dieters.

Physically, the men experienced a drop in their metabolic rate, as well as lowered body temperatures, breathing, and pulse rates. What I want to focus a bit more attention on, though, are the psychological and emotional responses. You may find yourself recognizing some of these.

Subjects showed a preoccupation with food, both during the starvation and rehabilitation phase. They would take a long time to eat their meals, they showed odd eating behaviors (chewing slowly, moving food around on their plates), and they felt tired and depressed. One extreme result was found in an individual who cut off three fingers! He wasn't sure if he had done this on purpose or by accident! Because of these men's constant preoccupation with food, they slowly became isolated and withdrawn.

Many of these psychological symptoms continued after the study was over. Published results report that subjects found themselves hoarding food whenever they could and binging whenever they had a chance. They experienced personality changes. According to one write-up of this study, one gentleman found it difficult to date his girlfriend because all he could think about was the food. Where were they going? What were they going to eat? Would he be able to get the kind of food he liked?

Do you recognize any of these symptoms? Do any of them apply to you?

While these young men volunteered for an experiment to aid in the war effort, how many of us have volunteered to participate in similar behavior as we wage our own war with weight?

This study was done under carefully controlled, carefully monitored conditions. But every day thousands of women consume less than 1500 calories per day and make themselves run miles every day—and unfortunately, these conditions are uncontrolled and the women feel out of control.

The point of describing the above study was to show you how healthy, young, *male* volunteers, when put into severe dieting situations, experience the exact psychological and emotional (as well as physical) symptoms seen every day in women who choose to go on diets. Why do we volunteer to do this to ourselves? What can we do to stop this behavior?

Chapter 5: Fear of Food Freedom

Food freedom is simply how you feel when you are *At Peace with Food*. You feel as though you can make the food choices you want without concern about what you *should* be eating, or what is better or worse. You make choices with complete freedom because you trust yourself and your body. Of course, sometimes you will choose that candy, those cookies, the piece of pie. But you know that you will also be able to balance those choices with the foods that provide the nutrients your body needs, not just the foods you want. And that's what it is about—balance. Balance, and freedom.

But people have a fear of this food freedom. Why? Think about it. What happens when I tell you that you have unconditional permission to eat what you want when you want, because you are in the process of learning to distinguish between the different types of hungers that are in your life? I bet your first response is "I can't do that!"

Why not?

Because you are afraid you will lose control. This is the response I hear most often: "I can't do that because once I start I will never be able to stop." You're afraid that once you start eating, you will gain so much weight that you'll never be able to lose it, and you'll hate yourself.

In short, you don't trust yourself, right?

Giving yourself unconditional permission to eat can be a truly liberating experience, honest! But yes, it is also scary. You probably *will* gain weight once you let go of the fear, the proverbial shackles that have been forcing you to go on diets for so many years.

Allow yourself to experience this fear, and then let it go.

Once the fear is gone, you'll find yourself with a lot of "space" to fill in with so many other activities. Once you've stopped being afraid of what you may choose to eat and start trusting yourself to make the right choices for *you*, you may discover a whole new way of looking a life. Once you've stopped being afraid you can start finding new ways to fill your life. You can concentrate on friendships, activities you've ignored because you didn't want to be seen, books you can read that aren't about the latest fad diet.

Honor Your Hunger

This doesn't mean putting your hunger feelings up on a pedestal and ignoring them. Rather, you should learn to listen to what your body is telling you. As you learn to become *At Peace with Food*, you discover what your hunger is about, and you learn to feed it appropriately.

Yet another of the ways dieting fails you is that it causes you lose what is called "hunger awareness." There are many different types of hunger (and you know this). When you are dieting, though, you have to ignore all forms of hunger because you're depriving yourself of food. You forget about all the different ways to be hungry, and to feed hunger.

Is there a grumbling in your stomach telling you it's time? Yes, it may have been more than three hours since breakfast, but if you're not hungry at noon, do you really need to eat lunch then?

So instead of dieting, learn to listen to yourself. Feelings of physical hunger occur when our bodies needs to eat: our glucose or glycogen stores have gone down, our blood sugars are dropping, and we need nourishment (which may be a peanut butter sandwich and milk, a steak, or fruit and cheese—and then, perhaps, that piece of chocolate). If we only ate when our bodies were in this state, then we probably wouldn't be overweight. But we eat for a whole host of other reasons. We are feeding a hunger, we just don't know what that hunger is.

Let's spend some time figuring out what that other hunger is, and what we can do about it.

One exercise I have clients do is *listen*. I tell them to learn to listen to themselves. Sometimes I say, "Put your hand over your mouth. Are you Mouth Hungry?" In other words, are you hungry because you want to taste something? Perhaps that coffee cake you smelled as you went by the bakery this morning just made you start salivating. That is what I call Mouth Hungry.

If that doesn't ring a bell, I say, "Put your hand over your heart." This indicates another type of hunger. Are you "Heart Hungry?" This type of hunger means your heart hurts; you are emotionally hungry. Perhaps you need a hug. Maybe you need to punch someone. (Though I'm not a particular advocate of this type of feeding response, I do recognize it as a reality.) Maybe you need a bath. Or perhaps at this particular moment, you are Heart Hungry for a chocolate brownie, just to treat yourself.

Then I say, "Put your hand over your stomach." This is the physical hunger—not just stomach grumbling; several hours may have passed since your last meal and you have been too busy to realize it. If you can take a moment to figure out that *this* is your hunger, then hopefully you will feed it appropriately with a meal that you will enjoy.

You see? They are many different types of hunger, and you need to sit down and discover for yourself what those different hungers are, when they occur, and what *you* need to do to feed them appropriately. If it's a chocolate brownie (yes, I do have a chocolate theme), then by all means, have one. But also take some time to eat and enjoy it. Maybe you'll discover that you can fill this hunger with only half a brownie, and you can save the rest for later.

If you discover a different type of hunger occurring, then figure out how to feed it. Maybe you need to take some time to be by yourself, take a bath, or visit a friend and ask for a hug. If you're emotionally hungry and this is what will "fill you up," do it. Not all our hungers need to be satisfied with calories. That is a big part of becoming *At Peace with Food*: learning when your body needs food but also being at peace when your body doesn't need it. Discover the right type of nourishment, and consume it appropriately.

Good and Bad Foods: Don't Make Me Want to Shoot You

Just as I'm tired of people saying they've been "bad" because of what they've eaten, I'm also tired of them telling me they have eaten something "bad." I've already described what I want to do with those poor folks (but I won't, because I happen to like my freedom, food and otherwise). But you *must* learn to remove these labels from your food choices.

For example, if you're a diabetic, you may have been told never to eat sugar. But in truth, when diabetics haven't eaten for a long time or have taken too much medication, sugar may be the only thing that saves them. When blood sugars drop to a dangerously low level, a diabetic can faint or go into a coma. I have recommended that diabetics carry small tubes of cake icing around for that quick sugar boost in case of this dire situation. The pure dose of sugar (or sucrose) helps their blood sugars go up quickly. Then, of course, they must follow this up with eating food that will prevent blood sugars from dropping again—usually a sandwich with protein and fat, or cheese and crackers. The point is, for a diabetic in this situation, sugar may save a life.

So stop labeling foods as good and bad, and learn to think of them as foods you want or don't want. As you learn to understand and trust yourself, as you learn about the different types of hungers you experience, you will learn how to feed them with the correct nourishment.

Learn to figure out what you really want to eat, then allow yourself to eat it. Allow yourself to enjoy your food choices, whether you choose a cookie or a carrot stick (and yes, sometimes you may indeed choose a carrot stick). As you build trust with your ability to make choices, you'll be able to take care of yourself and make the choices that are good—for you.

Chapter 6: The Food Court of Law

When you decide you want to have that luscious piece of pie for dessert, in those brief moments between thinking you have to have it and then choosing it, you have put yourself in the position of being on trial. I call this the "Food Court of Law."

In those few moments you feel like you're in a situation in which you are going to be judged; there is someone out there watching you, listening as you present your arguments in favor of making this choice.

You, the defendant: Your Honor, I have been "good" today. I didn't eat breakfast or lunch, and now I have earned this pie.

Prosecutor: Your Honor, the defendant is starving herself and thinks of this pie as a reward for her behavior. Not only that, but once she eats the pie, she'll get fat and ugly and no one will want to look at her. She is incapable of making healthy food choices and should never be allowed to eat pie again.

Judge: I decide in favor of the prosecution. You cannot be trusted to eat "good" foods. And if you order this dessert, I will find you:

GUILTY, GUILTY, GUILTY.

Where has all this come from? Society? The media? Our parents? All the above? Regardless of how it started, we have a whole demographic of people (primarily women) who feel they are committing a crime by deciding to have dessert, or a large roast beef sandwich, and that they must be prosecuted because of this want. If we eat what we really want to, we think we'll be caught by the food police, tried in the Food Court of Law, and sentenced to Food Prison, where we serve our term waiting for the next diet to tell us what to eat.

But *we* have created this court. *We* have decided that others can judge us. When we are defensive about the food we eat, when we cannot enjoy our meals (and snacks and desserts) because we feel like we're breaking some law, we find ourselves on the defensive. It is a miserable place to be, isn't it, always looking over your shoulder afraid someone is watching you eat?

Stop listening to those voices in your head, on the television, in the hair salon. Stop listening to those skinny people who ask, "How can you possibly eat that? You know it's bad for you!"

At the risk of sounding repetitive (again), I must reiterate that only by learning to trust ourselves will we be able to stop going to court.

Perhaps we need to think of ourselves as "food mediators." We are not going to judge ourselves anymore! Of course, we cannot turn off the television, the radio, or the folks at the hair salon— but we can learn to filter the material we hear. As we become *At Peace with Food*, we learn to enjoy food, we make choices we want, and the members of the Food Court can no longer prosecute us.

Normal Eating: It's Time for a Change

Once we've fired the Food Court of Law, we can learn to eat normally. But for many of us, it has been so long since we have allowed ourselves to feel hungry and enjoy food that we have lost all sense of how to associate *normal* with *eating*.

Ellyn Satter is a wonderful author of many books on eating behaviors, and I have learned a lot from her about what normal eating really involves. For example, do you realize it's normal to go to the table hungry and eat until you are full? While that's what we like to think we're doing, most of the time we wait until we are starving (as opposed to simply hungry), or else we eat because the clock says it is time for a meal.

It's also normal to overeat sometimes and under-eat at others. This can be eating three meals a day, or four to five times a day (what I call "mini meals and maxi snacks"). Sometimes it's grazing.

Regardless of what form it takes, however, normal eating includes eating when you're happy and giving yourself permission to eat because you are sad, or bored, or because the smell of fresh chocolate chip cookies is too wonderful to pass up.

Normal eating is learning to trust yourself and your body to, over time, make up for what you might consider to be "mistakes" in your food choices. But since you are allowed to make these choices, they are no longer considered mistakes; they are simply choices. Yes, you have days when you overeat, but if you learn to trust yourself you'll find that those days balance out with the days when you're not eating as much.

When this starts happening, you discover that eating begins to take its place as only *one* of the important areas of your life. You stop thinking about food all the time; it's just something that you now enjoy and have fun doing.

Behavior Chain

Are you familiar with the phrase "a chain is only as strong as its weakest link"? It can be applied to many situations—for example, a business is only as powerful as its weakest employee. When the competition finds that weak link, it can break the business.

We are going to apply this phrase in a positive manner and learn to use it to improve eating behaviors by breaking links in the chain that keeps us stuck in that Food Prison.

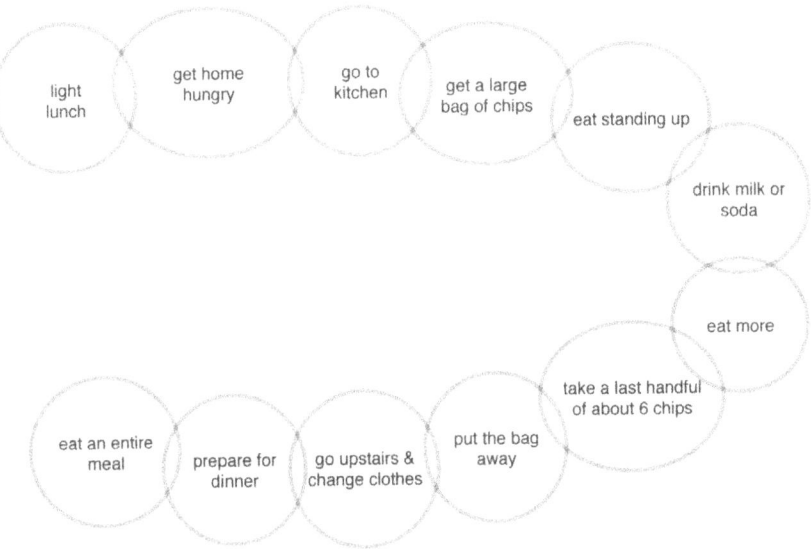

Above is an example of a Behavior Chain. Look carefully at the different links and let's pick a few and try to break them.

The first link, "eat a light lunch," leads to "get home hungry." How can we break that link? Perhaps by eating a larger lunch. If your lunch only consists of yogurt and carrot sticks and you don't get home for another five hours, you're going to be famished!

How about a tuna fish sandwich along with those carrot sticks and yogurt? Or if that's too much at one time, have the sandwich for lunch and save the rest for a snack about two hours later.

Let's look at the next two links. Perhaps on this day you didn't remember to bring a larger lunch. You get home and go directly into the kitchen to get a large bag of chips. How to break this link? Perhaps you could go directly to your bedroom instead, lie down for a few minutes, and relax. If you aren't really "stomach hungry" and just need to rest, then you have fed yourself appropriately.

But if that doesn't work and you go directly to the kitchen, perhaps you can find something less tempting than the large bag of chips. Perhaps this is when the yogurt would work. Or, instead of buying the large bag of chips, buy small bags that have a definite beginning, middle, and end. Instead of diving into that large bag and eating the equivalent of four small ones, you can simply take one small bag and eat the whole thing.

Do you see what we're going with this? We are going through each link of the chain and making "link breakers." Under these circumstances, breaking the link is a good thing and isn't going to destroy the "company."

Perhaps your "homework" for today can be picking one or two of our unbroken links and figuring out how to break them!

But remember, there will be days when you've gone through each link and find that nothing works—you are still going to eat. When you're *At Peace with Food*, you know that this type of behavior is fine, because over time it becomes the exception, not the rule.

Chapter 7: Three Rules of Thumb

Here are my three "rules of thumb" when it comes to being *At Peace with Food*. Perhaps *guidelines* might be better than *rules*, though, because once you start down the road of rules, you begin with the "shoulds."

(But "guidelines of thumb" just doesn't have the same ring, does it?)

1. Don't give up your favorite foods, just try to bring down the amount.

This is perhaps one of my most favorite phrases for teaching folks about food and eating. It's about portion size, ladies and gentlemen, not deprivation and starvation. There's no reason to eliminate the foods you enjoy from your life just because you're trying to lose weight. That only makes you want to eat them even more!

I know if someone told me I could never eat chocolate chip cookies again, I'd have to go out, buy a large bag, and consume the entire purchase, probably in one sitting. Yes, it would make me sick, but who has the right to tell me what I can and cannot eat?

When you are *At Peace with Food*, you may discover that two chocolate chip cookies satisfy your hunger. If you choose to eat more, though, it's okay, because you're learning to balance those cookies with other choices you're discovering you like, including "healthy foods" like fruits and vegetables. You are learning balance.

Once a colleague and I held a workshop on being *At Peace with Food*. We asked participants to bring one of their forbidden foods with them, and we would include the food as part of the workshop. We talked about all the topics you've been reading about, and eventually, after what perhaps seemed like an impossible amount of time, we asked our folks to take out their foods. We discussed with them why they felt these foods were "bad" (and I didn't shoot anyone). Eventually we all shared the foods and enjoyed them tremendously.

The next day when we got together for the second part of the workshop, we asked what everyone had eaten when they had dinner the previous night. Let me tell you: without exception, each person had chosen foods that would have made their mothers proud! And these choices were made not out of guilt, or "should," but because of choice! Folks had picked salads, broiled foods, and vegetables because they knew that these foods were what their bodies wanted.

You will learn this as well. When you're able to give up that fear of losing control, you'll discover that you're easily able to include the foods you love but that you will be able to eat them in smaller portions. Why? Because you've learned to taste and enjoy these foods, and you will discover that having given yourself unconditional permission to eat, smaller amounts satisfy your hunger.

2. Don't eat around your craving, figure out what you want, and go for it!

Have you ever found yourself hungry, food hungry (you've gone through those steps and decided what you really want to do is *eat food*), but you don't know what you want to eat? So you stand in front of the open refrigerator, freezer, food closet, whatever, and just start eating. You eat whatever you find yet are not satisfied. And what happens? You eat more than you ever wanted to and you feel full—but not content. And, you feel guilty.

Why is that?

Probably it's because you didn't take enough time to figure out what you really wanted to eat.

As you learn to listen to your body, you learn about what you really want—and the figuring out how to feed your hunger takes much less time. How do you learn to listen to your body? You learn your feelings of fullness and hunger. The next time you sit down and eat a meal, think about your feelings of fullness. Listen to your body, to your mind, to your throat, to your stomach. Are you full early in the meal? Are you full later in the meal? It's not going to be the same each time you sit down to eat, but eventually you'll find out what's right for you and learn to stop eating when you've reached your fullness level.

Try stopping yourself one third of the way through your meal. How do you feel? Are you okay? Do you feel hungry? Deprived? Do you continue to eat because you should? Remember what I said: don't *should* on yourself!

What are those feelings you find yourself experiencing? Are you still hungry? Are you anxious? Are you afraid you may overeat later if you don't finish everything on your plate? You *can* finish what you are eating; you are simply learning how to listen and not to judge (you are being a mediator, right? A nonjudgmental one). Eventually you will learn to tune into what it is you are hungry for, and you will feed yourself appropriately.

You've given yourself permission to eat, so now just take a few extra minutes and figure out exactly what food you want. Think about what you really want. Are you hungry for the crispness of potato chips? The sweetness of chocolate sauce (yes, I have heated up the hot fudge and just had that because it is what I wanted!), the texture of ice cream (not the fake stuff, the real stuff)? Do you want something hot? Cold? Sweet? Salty?

As you learn to listen to your hunger, you'll find you are also learning to feed it appropriately. Take a few extra minutes to discover what you really want, because I promise you, the food will taste so much better when it's what you *know* you want. Stop eating around your hunger and figure it out! You are learning so much about yourself, your cravings, your different hungers. And the most wonderful part of this discovery is that when you have made this time to take care of yourself, as you become *At Peace with Food* you will realize smaller portions are often all you really wanted, really needed, to be satisfied.

3. Stop all that non-charitable giving

You are learning how to listen to your body, to listen to your hunger. Perhaps you haven't quite gotten to the point where you can apply these new skills to food because something is still holding you back. What is it?

Is it that fear of losing control we discussed earlier? Is it the guilt? Thank you again, Erma Bombeck, for reminding us "guilt is the gift that keeps on giving." The question is *why*.

Okay, you're only human. It's taken many years for you to get to this point, so you're not going to unlearn behaviors in just a few days. But you are starting.

My experience with people who talk about feeling guilty is that all guilt does is make them overeat even more. They figure, *I've already overeaten. I've already done something bad.* Oh no, not that "bad" again! And there you are, being your own judge and jury, condemning yourself. What happens? You decide, *I've already started down this path. I'm already on a roll of bad behavior, so I'm going to stay on it.*

As a matter of fact, I recently had a conversation with a friend who had lost twenty pounds by the end of last year. In the first six months of the New Year, she started putting the weight back on. She wanted to talk to me about it, so I asked what happened. She told me she was stressed at work and had stopped walking. She felt that the combination of all these behaviors was too overwhelming to even start to make a difference. She had started with the "shoulds"—I *should* be more active, I *should* enjoy my food, I *should* slow down. She felt she could no longer simply be *At Peace with Food*, she had to *work* at being *At Peace with Food*. She felt if she couldn't do everything right at one time, she might as well not try. She felt guilty and couldn't stop herself.

As we continued to talk, I asked her to try what I want you to try: imagine what it's like giving up the guilt. Imagine how you'd feel if you looked at that bowl of ice cream and said, "I feel like eating it and I am going to eat it all." Imagine *not* saying, "I'm bad because I like ice cream." Imagine *not* saying, "I need to eat more because I've done something bad."

Just take a few moments and think about what it would be like to give up that guilt. Take a pen and piece of paper and write down some of these feelings, okay?

When you allow yourself the liberation from guilt, when you release yourself from these feelings, suddenly you find there is a whole lot of other room inside your mind to enjoy life, to enjoy food, and to feel good about yourself. Once you experience these wonderful feelings, you are beginning to experience the benefits of being *At Peace with Food*. And when you are *At Peace with Food*, you don't have guilt, you don't have anger or self-condemnation. You are enjoying your life. You enjoy the food you choose and you have created a relationship you can build on. Your relationship with food is now going to become one of enjoyment and deliciousness!

Chapter 8: About Weight Control

Because I know you're interested, I want to give you some basic information about weight control. I'm more concerned about you developing a new and healthy relationship with food, but I want to make sure your basics of losing weight are correct.

And here it is: simple, yet one of the most complicated statements for folks concerned about losing weight.

Weight is a balance of intake and expenditure.

That's it. What it means takes a little longer, but you need to know it.

By intake and expenditure, I mean calories. In my field we refer to calories as energy. This is different from the advertising you may see for energy drinks or pills, vitamins, and the like that promise to give you energy. When you have your coffee and vitamins in the morning and suddenly feel energetic, it's not the pills; it's the caffeine.

Weight is a balance of calorie intake versus calorie expenditure, or calories used, by the body. Where do these calories come from?

Energy Intake

Intake refers to the calories in the foods we consume, from proteins, carbohydrates, and fats. While I will give you some more guidelines about healthy eating in the next chapter, I'd like you to start thinking about what you do with the calories you consume.

You may hear that certain foods are "better" than others, and we've already discussed what I want to do with folks who talk about "good versus bad" foods. But in the end, I like to think that *flavor* is the first consideration when making food choices. If flavor is not considered, then eating becomes a chore.

I remember working with an eating disorder program when I first moved to Massachusetts. I worked in a locked ward for people with anorexia and bulimia. One of my jobs was to make sure that the anorexic patients were at least being served enough calories. I wasn't in charge of making sure they ate the food—that belonged to the behavioral specialists. But I do remember having many conversations with patients who just didn't want to eat, part of their pathology. So I had to remind them that they weren't well; as a matter of fact, they were very sick. I told them they needed to look at food as though it were medicine; they might not like the way it tasted but they needed it in order to get better.

You don't need this advice—you need the opposite. You need to learn to *enjoy* food again; and as we've discussed, once you've learned to give up guilt, you will find yourself enjoying many foods you once thought you *had* to eat. Yes, they may be full of nutrients, but that becomes a side issue—extra credit, if you will. You eat these foods because they taste good.

In addition to learning to enjoy your food, make time to eat. Try not to eat on the run. I realize that in this day and age it is very difficult to sit down and have a meal. But when you make time, take a few minutes to sit down and think about what you are eating, you'll find you're more able to appreciate food choices.

Have you ever sat down in front of the TV set with a bowl of chips? Or gone to the movies and bought the large popcorn? Are you sitting there for a few minutes and suddenly notice there is no more food? This is what I call "unconscious eating." You've consumed a large amount of food without ever having a chance to enjoy it.

I went to a workshop on "creating health" many years ago. It's a wonderful title, but I'm not really sure I remember everything the woman discussed or if I'm a healthier person today because of the class. However, I do remember her talking about paying attention to eating food. She described how once or twice a year all the educators get together for a weekend to learn the latest information on this topic so they can go back to their communities and give more classes. She talked about how wonderful the food is at these events, and how everyone always eats a lot. But she also talked about how at one meal during the weekend, people eat in silence. As a result, people always leave food on their plate!

This has always stayed with me. It made me realize how much eating we do without ever thinking about it. It may be impossible for you to sit down and think about all your meals, but it certainly could be a goal to consume one meal a week in silence.

"You people don't eat food, you *inhale* it!" my mother used to tell us. She would spend at least half an hour preparing meals and we would finish them in less than five minutes. Of course, there were four of us girls, along with my parents, and we were always talking and eating; but it did seem to go fast. And so my mother would lament our inability to chew our food.

Take a breath. When you do get to sit down and eat, take a deep breath before you start. Just relax, put your hands on the table (or in your lap), and take a moment before you begin to eat. Try to take that moment at a different time from when you try to have a meal in silence. See how each affects your behavior.

Energy Expenditure

This is a bit more complicated, but it refers to the calories your body uses throughout the day. When I teach energy expenditure to my students, I divide it into three categories:

1. Basal metabolic rate—the calories burned by "just being." Basal metabolism burns about 60-65 percent of the calories you consume. This energy is used for what is often referred to as "involuntary activities" such as breathing, nerve impulses, even blinking your eyes. This is a huge amount of energy, isn't it? But your body wants to survive, and it does so by using all this energy for all these activities.

2. Thermic effect of food— the calories used to digest, absorb, and metabolize the food you eat. This uses about 5-10 percent of the calories you consume. I love this particular category, because it always brings up the "celery" question—you know, is it true it takes more calories to eat celery than is actually in the celery itself?

   And now you know the answer: no. If a piece of celery has ten calories, then one calorie is used (one calorie being 10 percent of the total calories found in a stick of celery). However, I think the more important question is why would anyone want to eat that much celery?

3. Activity—exercise, also known as "voluntary activities" in the body. This is the one component of energy expenditure you can control. You can increase or decrease your activity, thus increasing or decreasing the amount of calories burned during what is officially known as "muscle contraction."

    Physical activity uses about 20-25 percent of the calories we consume. This is a very important component of energy expenditure, and one that many people hate. Telling people to increase their exercise is probably one of the most difficult parts of my job.

Experience has shown me that, believe it or not, losing weight is easy. Keeping it off is what is hard. And I've learned that folks who've made exercise (or what we will soon be referring to as "activity") part of their lives are able to take the weight off and keep it off.

This is such an important topic that the next section is devoted to learning how to be…

At Peace with Exercise

When we lived in State College, Pennsylvania, my husband and I were friends with a lovely couple we'll call Joe and Irene.

We used to go walking with them in the hills of central Pennsylvania. These walks could be quite strenuous, but they were always fun and good exercise.

However, Joe and Irene would tell anyone who would listen that they absolutely hated hiking and refused to consider going on one. While they refused to use the word *hiking*, however, they would sometimes *walk* for an entire day.

Why was this terminology so important to them? They felt that "hiking" implied fancy expensive waterproof mountain boots, hydration packs, trekking poles, and freeze dried food. All they wanted to do was take some water and a few snacks and be off for the day.

I always think of this couple when I talk to clients about exercise. For some reason, to many people the word *exercise* implies buying a membership to an expensive club, going to a fancy store, and purchasing athletic garb to wear on the machines. Don't forget the headband to catch sweat and, of course, the most expensive vitamin/mineral flavored water.

The concept of regular exercise is quite daunting for many people. It implies hours each day and dollars most people can't afford. It creates pictures of people climbing up and down (in place) on machines in the club windows—you know you've seen them as you walk down the street.

If you're a club member who really enjoys what you're doing, then bravo. I may even be jealous of you. I certainly encourage folks with the resources to go ahead and join. But only if this is what you really want to do, not what you think you *should* do.

For the others, however, I try to find a happy medium. Instead of the word *exercise*, I start with the phrase "increasing your activity." To me, a body in motion as opposed to a body at rest is *active*. Using those large muscle groups, like the ones found in your legs, takes a lot of energy; and that energy is what burns calories. When these muscles are used for longer periods of time, your body burns more calories.

My preferred activity is simply walking. While it may eventually require a more expensive sneaker (or "walking shoes" as I like to call them), a regular sturdy sneaker or shoe is fine for beginning a walking program. I encourage my clients to start walking five minutes, three times a week. Usually they say, "But that's nothing." I always ask, "So what's stopping you?"

Once they do this for two weeks, I suggest increasing the time to ten minutes, three times a week, then adding five minutes every two weeks until they are walking thirty or forty minutes three times a week—and lastly, adding an additional day so they are walking a total of forty to forty-five minutes four times a week.

Here's the "program" I give to folks:

WHEN	HOW LONG	HOW OFTEN
Weeks 1-2	5 minutes	3x/week
Weeks 3-4	10-15 minutes	3x/week
Weeks 5-6	20-25 minutes	3x/week
Weeks 7-8	30-35 minutes	3x/week
Weeks 9-10	40-45 minutes	3x/week
Weeks 11-12	40-45 minutes	3-4x/week

This doesn't have to be all at one time, either, especially if you don't have that large a block free. Studies suggest that walking ten minutes three or four times a day may be just as beneficial as a single forty-five-minute walk. Use the "talk, don't whistle" formula for measuring intensity, meaning that if you can whistle while you walk, you are moving too slowly. If you can't talk while you're walking, your pace is too fast.

What do you think? If you start at five minutes three times a week, in three months you could be walking forty-five minutes three or four times a week! The idea is to start slowly, be realistic, and enjoy yourself.

Remember, exercise—oops, I mean, being active—isn't a punishment. Don't think of it as something you are doing *to* yourself; think of it as something you are doing *for* yourself.

Many times I am asked, "What's the best exercise to do?" The answer is actually another question: what do you *like* to do? If you've heard that running is the "best" exercise but you hate to run, that doesn't bode well for setting realistic, attainable goals, does it? If you were told you had to get up an hour early and run three miles in order to improve your health, you'd hit the snooze and roll over in bed when the alarm went off. Or perhaps you'd do it once or twice because that's what you *should* to do. But sooner rather than later you'd get tired of feeling forced to do something you don't like, and you would feel guilty because of the "shoulds." Soon after that, anger and self-doubt would rear their ugly heads and you'd find yourself heading down a familiar path that doesn't lead in a good direction.

The other popular question is "what is the best time of day to exercise?" To be honest, I don't know. I'm sure there are studies that give recommendations, but I don't use those results in my practice. My recommendation? Whenever you have the time. If you can't get up early but have time later in the day, that's when you walk (or whatever you like to do). If you work in an office and can take short breaks during the day, that's your time to move. Again, it's an individual decision, an individual choice. Find a time that works for you, and that is the best time.

Figuring out what's realistic for you allows you to be successful, and you can build on that success. You need to set small, attainable goals and increase them as you are ready. What I've listed above are guidelines, not rules, so you can't "break" them, okay?

When you're honest with yourself about your goals, you learn about your limits. Understand that when you experience aches and pains, your body is telling you that you may be moving too quickly. Don't let your ego get ahead of your ability! That's why the guidelines I've suggested may seem ridiculously slow. But it's better for you to take your time reaching your goal than to rush and injure yourself, making it impossible for you to be involved in *any* activity.

Be flexible. Know that some days you're not going to be able to meet those goals, but remember: there's always the next day.

It's progress that counts. You are building on *your* goals, not anyone else's.

The bottom line? Whether you're a hiker or a walker, a club member or a solitary biker, words don't matter. Staying active does.

Chapter 9: Learning to Be a Healthy Eater

I would be remiss as a health care provider if I didn't at least review some of the basics of making healthy choices. For you to be able to make healthy food choices, you must have a healthy relationship with the foods you eat. This is why I've purposefully waited until the end to address this, because I believe that learning about yourself and your relationship with food is more important than giving factual information about good nutrition. All the advice in the world is useless if you haven't learned about *why* you make your choices.

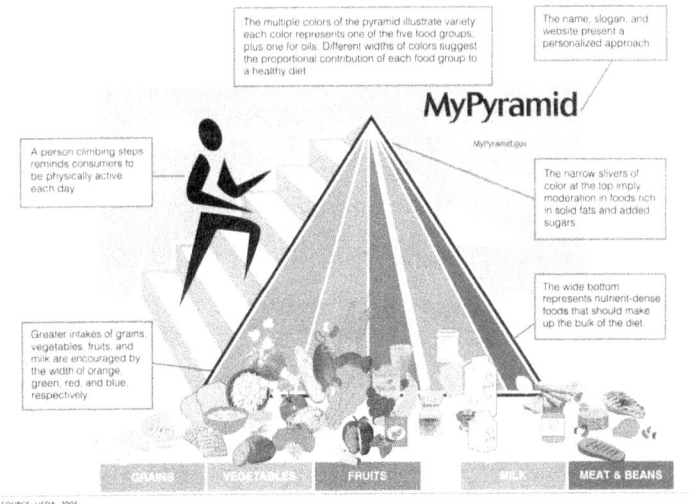

SOURCE: USDA, 2005

Let me introduce you to a wonderful Web site: www.mypyramid.gov. This is an interactive site that uses Web technology to make it easier for you to design your own personal eating plan. It came out in January of 2005 and was designed to replace the Food Guide Pyramid.

This new program takes into account what we've been saying throughout this book: everyone is different, and we all have different nutritional needs. Using www.mypyramid.gov, you can learn how to make healthy food choices as well as plan a physical activity program that is based on your personal needs. It's not supposed to provide for people in need of therapeutic diets, though; if you have diabetes or kidney problems, for example, you need to see your health care provider and a registered dietitian for personalized help.

When you look at this site, you will learn (or relearn) many principles of nutrition. The different colors of the pyramid represent the different food groups, and the width of the "mini-pyramids" stands for how many servings you choose for a basic meal plan.

The different food groups include grains, vegetables, fruits, milk, meat and beans (you don't need to eat a twelve-ounce steak to get the protein your body needs), oils, and what they call "discretionary calories," or what I like to call "dessert."

It is recommended to choose *whole* grain breads and cereals. Remember, when you look at the label on a loaf of bread, "wheat flour" doesn't mean "whole wheat." Processed white flour is technically still a type of wheat flour, so you need to look more closely at the ingredients. Whole grain breads and cereals provide you with fiber, which is a type of carbohydrate your body doesn't digest but may help reduce symptoms of constipation ("keep you regular") and may help lower blood cholesterol.

Vegetables and fruits are excellent sources of fiber, along with vitamins, minerals, and water. I like to tell my clients to "eat from the rainbow," a phrase I learned from one of my *Food and Health Communications* handouts. This means the more color you add to your diet, the healthier your food choices. At the end of the day, instead of thinking, *Did I eat my five servings of fruits?* try asking yourself, *What colors have I eaten?* and make that your way of adding variety to your choices.

As you become *At Peace with Food*, you will discover that foods you once thought of as "diet" foods, like apples, carrots, peaches, and celery, actually do taste good; and you will choose them because you want to, not because you *should*.

While protein, calcium, and vitamin D are the major nutrients found in dairy products, there are nondairy products out there for folks who are vegan or lactose intolerant. Soy beverages are one of the ways non-milk drinkers can ensure they get these nutrients, because the beverages are fortified with calcium and vitamin D.

Remember, it's not *what* you eat, it's *how much* you eat, especially when it comes to those of you who get your protein from animal products. While you can certainly get lean cuts of meat, it's still helpful to watch serving size. As you become *At Peace with Food*, you learn that smaller portions satisfy your needs, and it just so happens that those smaller portions still provide you with plenty of protein.

Should you be counting fat grams? Carbohydrate grams? No, you should be listening to your body, paying attention to your hunger, and feeding yourself appropriately.

When I first began working as an outpatient nutritionist in the Boston area, everyone was counting fat grams. One of my patients had lost perhaps twenty-five pounds using this method. But then she disappeared for a long time. One day she finally showed up, having gained back the weight she lost, plus some (sound familiar?). She sat next to my desk and said to me, "I remember the exact day it started. It was Easter, and I was looking at the box of Marshmallow Peeps, and I saw there was no fat—so I ate the whole box!"

That's what happens with counting fat grams! Fat-free doesn't mean calorie free! My patients began eating the entire box of fat-free brownies, or the entire half-gallon of fat-free frozen yogurt! If they had only listened to what they were truly craving and eaten a smaller portion of *real* ice cream, they would have saved themselves a lot of aggravation, and calories—and they probably would have enjoyed the taste more.

The same has happened with the low/no carbohydrate diets. Instead of eating real, delicious foods, people are choosing low carb breads, cookies, and cakes—looking at only the amount of carbohydrates in the food and not at what they are truly hungry for. Fortunately, this particular fad seems to be fading as well. Unfortunately, too many people still think there is a quick fix out there when it comes to diets and weight loss.

Flavor First

First and always, consider flavor when you make your food choices. As I said earlier, as you learn to listen to your hunger signals you may decide you want chocolate mousse ice cream. It's much better for you to have a portion of the real thing than to eat a half-gallon of fat-free chocolate yogurt. You may pay more for the "real" thing in terms of money, but as you listen to your body you will be satisfied with less; and the reduction in emotional and health costs will be well worth it.

The same goes for other low fat foods. I have occasionally recommended certain low fat cheeses to my clients, but only because I believe they taste as good as the full flavor product.

Quality of Life Is at the Top of the List

Don't let your last thought be *I should have had the cheesecake.*

This may be another way of saying, "Flavor first." Having discussed the pitfalls of setting unrealistic goals of eating the foods you don't like because you are afraid to eat the ones you love, of dragging yourself out of bed too early because you *should* be exercising before you leave for work, I want you to remember this: you only set yourself up for failure.

When you decide you absolutely cannot choose the sugar free sorbet instead of the lemon meringue pie, then you better make sure you love every bite. Take your time, find each and every taste bud on your tongue, and make sure this delectable dessert works its way slowly through your mouth and down your throat. Don't you dare let yourself feel guilty about your decision.

Otherwise, all your efforts to becoming *At Peace with Food* are a waste of time.

Remember, quality of life is at the top of the list. I once had a diabetic patient who was truly miserable because she felt she could never eat pasta again. She loved her spaghetti with its marinara sauce along with a glass of red wine. But when she ate this type of meal in the evening, her blood sugars were very high the next morning. We tried several different strategies to help work this food into her meal plan, including increasing her activity in the evening. But it wasn't helping her blood sugars, so I suggested she talk to her primary care physician about making a small increase in her medication so she could eat the food she loved and still control her sugars. Guess what? It worked. Her blood sugars came down and she was much happier; the quality of her life rose dramatically and she had made changes she could live with, without sacrificing health or taste.

You need to consider these types of factors as you move forward with your plans to become *At Peace with Food*. If you find you cannot give up certain foods (and remember, I never said you needed to) or if you absolutely cannot reduce your portion of your favorite pie, then you need to evaluate your goals. If weight loss is your goal, consider other ways to reduce foods that are less important to you. Or find times to increase your activity levels. Don't forget about energy balance.

Perhaps being a size six isn't really necessary. If you can find the clothes you love in larger sizes and still eat the foods you like, then change those size goals. The idea is to stop worrying all the time about what you are going to eat, and start living.

The End, and a New Beginning: Making the Relationship Work

Becoming *At Peace with Food* is a journey that involves developing a new relationship with food. And then what I've mentioned before will start to happen to you: instead of being marked by frustration and disappointment, by fear and competition between you and the food you eat, food *will* take its place as one of the many activities in your life, along with family, friends, working, and being active. And, like these other activities, it *will be* pleasurable.

You must realize that your life isn't over just because you didn't lose those five, ten, or twenty pounds by the beginning of the summer or for your winter vacation. You have your whole life to learn to change your relationship with food. You have time, lots of it, to make this relationship with food a positive one.

Giving yourself unconditional permission to eat is a truly liberating experience. But remember, you need time to adjust to these new feelings. It took you many years to get to this point, so you're not going to change overnight.

We've discussed many different factors that have been part of your relationship with food, including fear, guilt, and that whole issue of "should." You are learning about yourself and how you developed this relationship with food. If you look at the different relationships in your life, you know that some of them are constantly changing while some of them are dependable and stay the same. Your relationship with food took time to develop, and it will take time to change. So take this time to learn about yourself, and let yourself be surprised with what you discover!

Good luck!

REFERENCES

Orbach, Susan. *Fat is a Feminist Issue II*. The Berkley Publishing Group, 1982.

'Obesity More Common in the South." <u>Washington Post</u>, July 18, 2008.

Gura, Trisha. *Lying in Weight: The Hidden Epidemic of Eating Disorders in Adult Women*. HarperCollins Publishers, 2007.

Chernin, Kim:.*The Obsession: Reflections on the Tyrrany of Slenderness*. Harper & Row, 1981.

Keyes, Ancel, et al. *The Biology of Human Starvation*. Univ of Minn. Press, 1950.

'Feeling Fine in '89,' Pennsylvania State University, 1989.